The Ultimate Vegan Air Fryer Cooking Guide

A Recipe Book to Prepare your Daily Meals

Samantha Attanasio

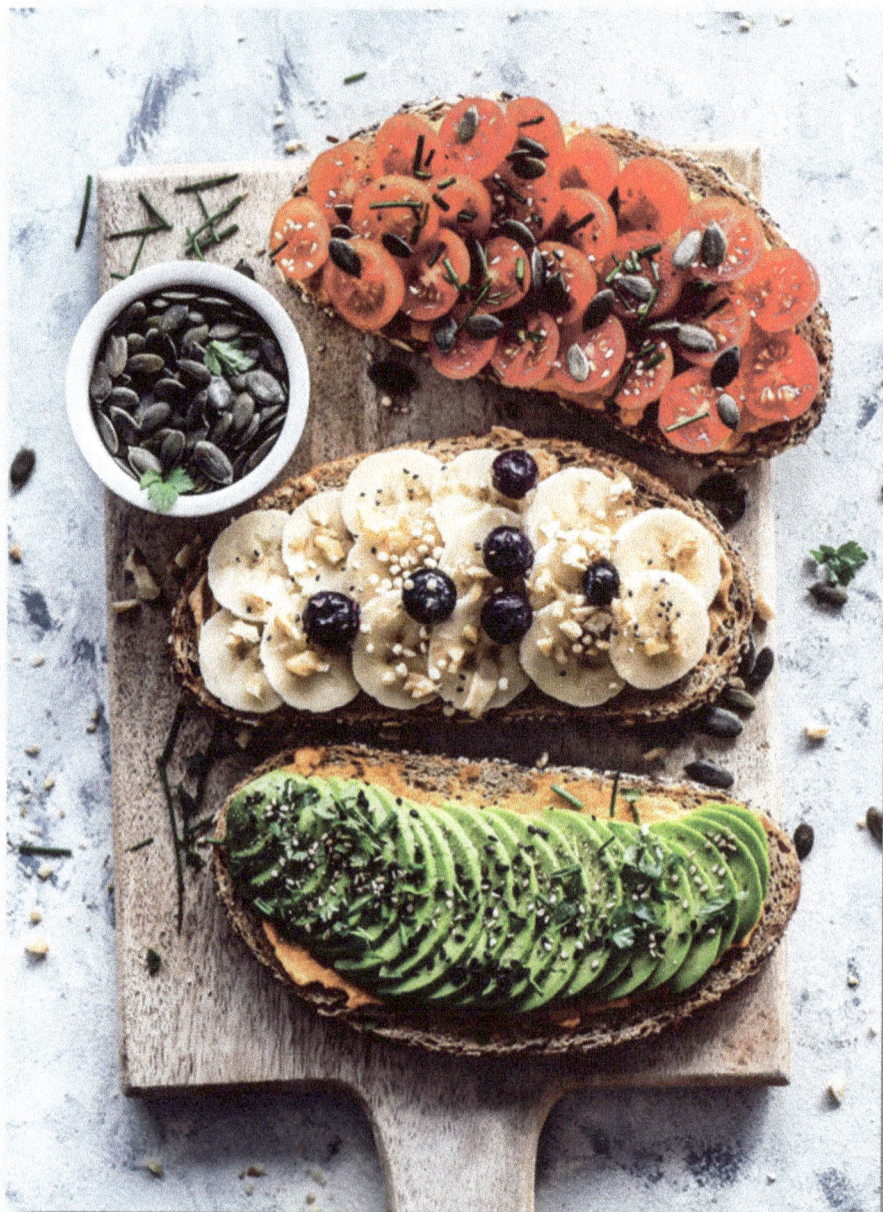

by reading this document, the reader agrees that under no circumstances is the author responsible for any losses, direct or indirect, which are incurred as a result of the use of information contained within this document, including, but not limited to, — errors, omissions, or inaccuracies.

Table of Contents

Vegetable

Savoury Chinese Cauliflower Rice

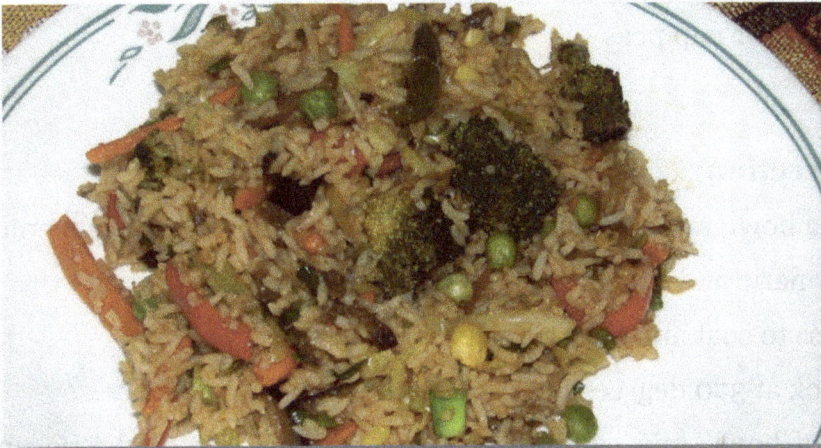

Preparation time: 10 minutes

Cooking time: 20 minutes

Servings: 4

Ingredients:

- Four tbsp. coconut aminos
- ½ block firm tofu, cubed
- 1 cup carrot, chopped
- ½ cup yellow onion, chopped

- One tsp. turmeric powder
- 3 cups cauliflower, riced
- 1½ tsp. sesame oil
- One tbsp. rice vinegar
- ½ cup broccoli florets, chopped
- One tbsp. ginger, minced
- Two garlic cloves, minced
- ½ cup peas

Direction:

In a bowl, mix tofu with two tbsp. coconut aminos, ½ cup onion, turmeric and carrot.

Toss to coat and then transfer into your air fryer.

Cook at 370 degrees F for 10 minutes, shaking halfway .

In a bowl, mix cauliflower rice with the rest of the coconut aminos, sesame oil, garlic, vinegar, ginger, broccoli and peas.

Stir and add to the tofu mix from the fryer.

Toss and cook everything at 370 degrees F for 10 minutes.

Divide between plates. Serve and enjoy!

Nutrition:

Energy (calories): 111 kcal

Protein: 6.56 g

Fat: 5.44 g

Carbohydrates: 11.34 g

Tasty Artichokes Dish

Preparation time: 5 minutes

Cooking time: 12 minutes

Servings: 4

Ingredients:

- Four big artichokes
- Salt and black pepper to taste
- Two tbsp. lemon juice
- ¼ cup olive oil
- Two tsp. balsamic vinegar
- One tsp. oregano, dried
- Two garlic cloves, minced

Direction:

Season artichokes with salt and pepper.

Now rub them with half of the oil and half of the lemon juice.

Next, put them in your air fryer and cook at 360 degrees F for 7 minutes.

In a bowl, mix these Ingredients the remaining oil, the lemon juice, with vinegar, salt, pepper, garlic and oregano and stir very well.

Divide artichokes between plates.

Drizzle the vinaigrette all over and serve them as a side dish.

Nutrition:

Energy (calories): 207 kcal

Protein: 5.68 g

Fat: 13.8 g

Carbohydrates: 19.74 g

Beet Salad

Preparation time: 10 minutes
Cooking time: 14 minutes
Servings: 4

Ingredients:

- Four beets, trimmed
- Two tbsp. balsamic vinegar
- A bunch of parsley, chopped
- Salt and black pepper to the taste
- One tbsp. extra-virgin olive oil
- One garlic clove, chopped
- Two tbsp. capers

Direction:

Put beets in your air fryer's basket and cook them at 360 degrees F for 14 minutes.

In a bowl, mix parsley with garlic, salt, pepper, olive oil and capers and stir very well.

Leave beets to cool down.

Now peel them, slice and put them in a bowl.

Next, add vinegar and the parsley mix.

Toss, divide between plates and serve as a side dish.

Nutrition:

Energy (calories): 33 kcal

Protein: 0.87 g

Fat: 1.68 g

Carbohydrates: 3.83 g

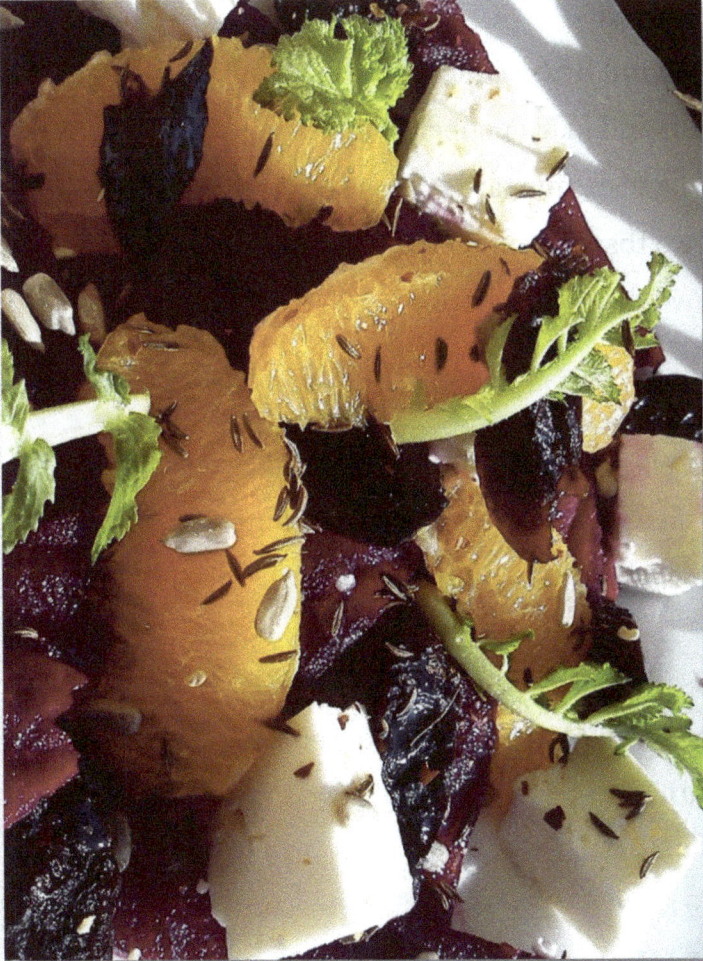

Creamy Brussels Sprouts

Preparation time: 3 minutes

Cooking time: 11 minutes

Servings: 4

Ingredients:

- 1 pound Brussels sprouts, trimmed
- Salt and black pepper to taste
- One tbsp. mustard
- Two tbsp. coconut cream
- Two tbsp. dill, chopped

Direction:

Put Brussels sprouts in your air fryer's basket.

Cook them at 350 degrees F for 10 minutes.

In a bowl, mix the cream with mustard, dill, salt and pepper and whisk.

Add Brussels sprouts and toss.

Divide between plates and best to serve as a side dish.

Nutrition:

Protein: 4.48 g

Fat: 3.09 g

Carbohydrates: 11.94 g

Yellow Lentil Mix

Preparation time: 10 minutes

Cooking time: 15 minutes

Servings: 2

Ingredients:

- 1 cup yellow lentils, soaked in water for 1 hour and drained
- One hot chilli pepper, chopped
- The 1-inch ginger piece, grated
- ½ tsp. turmeric powder
- One tsp. garam masala
- Salt and black pepper to taste
- Two tsp. olive oil
- ½ cup cilantro, chopped
- 1½ cup spinach, chopped
- Four garlic cloves, minced
- ¾ cup red onion, chopped

Direction:

In a pan that suites your air fryer, mix lentils with chilli pepper, ginger, turmeric, garam masala, salt, pepper, olive oil, cilantro, spinach, onion and garlic.

Toss, introduce in your air fryer.

Cook at 400 degrees F temperature for 15 minutes.

Divide lentil mix between plates. Serve and enjoy!

Nutrition:

Energy (calories): 115 kcal

Protein: 5.56 g

Fat: 5.01 g

Carbohydrates: 15.78 g

Veggie Lasagna

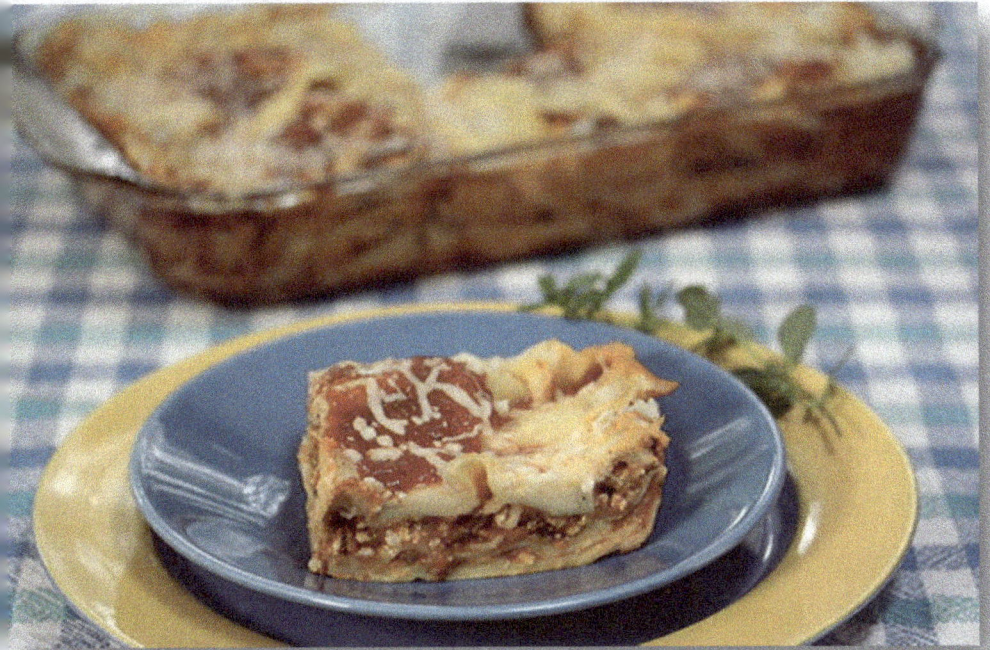

Preparation time: 10 minutes

Cooking time: 20 minutes

Servings: 4

Ingredients:

- 300 g / 0.66 lbs. zucchini

- One carrot
- 200 g / 0.44 lbs. tomatoes
- 200 g / 0.44 lbs. tofu
- 100 g / 0.4 cup water
- Four tsp. soy milk
- One tsp. black pepper
- One tsp. chilli pepper
- One tsp. cilantro
- One tsp. oregano
- One yellow onion

Directions

This veggie lasagna tastes even better than the lasagna with ground meat. Try it once, and you will want to eat it again and again. Remove the skin from the tomatoes. Take the bowl with hot water and put the tomatoes in it for 1 minute. Then remove the tomatoes from the water and peel them. Slice the tomatoes. Chop the tofu cheese. Peel the carrot and slice it. Peel the onion and chop it very roughly. Slice the zucchini with the help of a hand slicer. Preheat the air fryer to 190 C / 380 F. Take the big vessel and make the lasagna. Put the sliced zucchini in the bottom of the vessel, and then add little-chopped tofu. Then put the layer of tomatoes. Then add chopped onion. Then cover the mixture with the tofu again. Sprinkle the lasagna with oregano, cilantro, chilli and black peppers. Transfer it to the air fryer and close the lid. Cook it for 15 minutes. Serve it immediately.

Nutrition:

Caloric content 79 kcal

Proteins 6.2 grams

Fats 2.5 grams

Carbohydrates 10.4 grams

Onion Pie

Preparation time: 10 minutes

Cooking time: 35 minutes

Servings: 4

Ingredients:

- 150 g / 0.33 lbs. flour
- 50 g / 0.2 cup almond milk
- One tsp. salt
- 50 g / 0.2 cup water
- 300 g / 0.66 lbs. onion
- One tsp. olive oil
- 100 g / 0.22 lbs. tofu
- 50 g / 0.2 cup soy milk
- Four tomatoes

Directions:

Peel the onion and then chop it into tiny bits. Transfer the chopped onion to the big mixing bowl and sprinkle it with salt. Then chop the tofu cheese and add it to the mixing bowl too. Stir it gently till you get a homogenous mass. Take small tomatoes for this dish and cut them into two parts. Then leave the mixture with chopped onion and take another bowl and sift the flour in it. Add soy milk and almond milk. Take the hand mixer and mix the mass very carefully. Preheat the air fryer and set at 200 C / 390 F temperature. Meanwhile, take the pie tray and spray it with olive oil. Knead the dough very carefully. Then put it on the tray and make it flat. Transfer the onion mixture to the dough and add tomato halves. Take another vessel and pour water into it. Transfer the vessel with water to the air fryer and put the tray with pie in it. Close the lid and decrease the temperature to 180 C / 360 F and cook the pie for 20 minutes. Then open the lid and leave it for 10 minutes more. Enjoy!

Nutrition:

Caloric content 252 kcal

Proteins 8.5 grams

Fats 6.1 grams

Carbohydrates 42.3 grams

Veggie Pizza

Preparation time: 10 minutes

Cooking time: 20 minutes

Servings: 4

Ingredients:

- 100 g / 0.4 cup water
- One tsp. dried yeast
- One tsp. sugar
- Three tomatoes
- 100 g / 0.22 lbs. black olives
- One yellow zucchini
- 200 g / 0.44 lbs. tofu
- 100 g / 0.22 lbs. spinach
- Two tsp. dill
- Two tsp. parsley
- One tsp. tomato paste
- One sweet red pepper
- One onion
- 200 g / 0.44 lbs. flour

Directions:

Firstly make dough for pizza: take the big bowl and combine warm water with dried yeast. Stir it carefully till the yeast is dissolved. Then sprinkle the mass with sugar and stir it again. Sift the flour and add half of it to the mixture and stir it gently. Cover the mass with a towel and leave it in a warm place. Meanwhile, slice black olives and chop the tofu cheese. Slice the tomatoes and chop the red sweet pepper. Then peel the onion and chop it into small pieces. Chop the parsley and dill and combine them in the mixing bowl. Slice the zucchini. Preheat the air fryer and set to 200 C / 390 F. Meanwhile, remove the towel from the dough and stir it again gently. Add the other half of the dough and knead it. Then make the flat circle and transfer it to the tray. Put the tofu cheese in the bottom of the dough. Add sliced zucchini and onion. Then put red sweet pepper and tomatoes. Sprinkle the pizza with a mix of chopped parsley and dill. Transfer the pizza to the air fryer and cook it for 18 minutes. Remove the cooked pizza from the air fryer and serve it immediately. Enjoy!

Nutrition:

Caloric content 305 kcal

Proteins 12.7 grams

Fats5.8 grams

Carbohydrates 53.0 grams

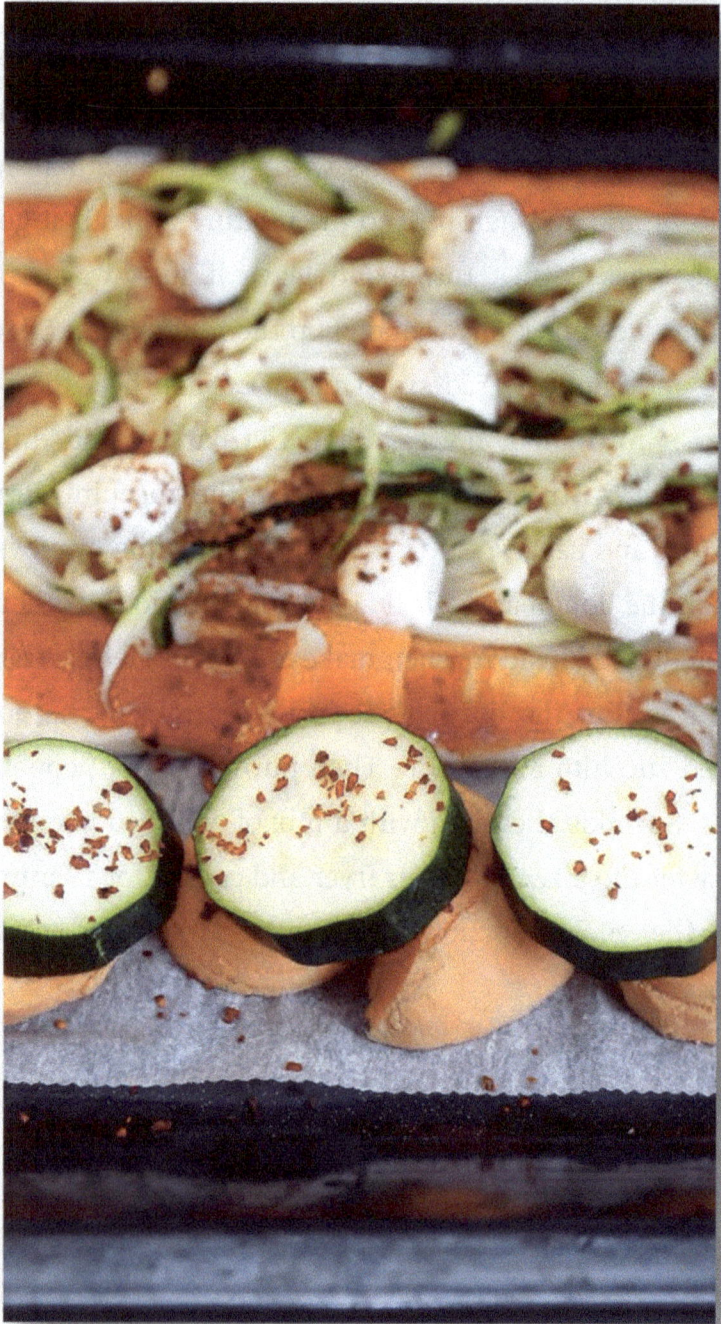

Festive Vegetable Stew

Preparation time: 10 minutes

Cooking time: 30 minutes

Servings: 4

Ingredients:

- 300 g / 0.66 lbs. tomatoes
- 200 g / 0.44 lbs. zucchini
- One onion
- Two sweet green peppers
- One sweet yellow pepper
- 100 g / 0.22 lbs. tomato paste
- 100 g / 0.4 cup almond milk
- One tsp. cilantro
- One tsp. chilli pepper
- 100 g / 0.22 lbs. leek
- 100 g / 0.22 lbs. lentils
- 300 g / 1.2 cup vegetables stock

Directions:

Chop the tomatoes into tiny pieces. Then slice the zucchini and cut it into two parts more. Remove the seeds from the sweet pepper and cut it into strips. Then cut each strip into two parts more. Chop the leek. Take the big bowl and combine all Ingredients in it. Stir it gently. Then add lentils to it and sprinkle the mass with the cilantro, chilli pepper, and tomato paste. Stir it carefully and leave it. Preheat the air fryer set at 200 C / 390 degrees F. Meanwhile, peel the onion and chop it roughly. Combine vegetable stock with almond milk and stir it. Then pour the liquid into the air fryer and add vegetable mass. Stir it gently with the help of the wooden spoon. Close the lid and cook it for 20 minutes. The lentils should absorb all water. Then remove the stew, chill it little and serve it immediately.

Nutrition:

Caloric content 247 kcal

Proteins 11.2 grams

Fats 7.1 grams

Carbohydrates 38.0 grams

Spinach Dish

Preparation time: 10 minutes

Cooking time: 0 minutes

Servings: 4

Ingredients:

- 200 g / 0.44 lbs. oatmeal flour
- 150 g / 0.6 cup water
- ½ tsp. baking soda
- 200 g / 0.44 lbs. spinach
- 100 g / 0.22 lbs. oatmeal
- One onion
- One tsp. olive oil
- One tsp. oregano
- One tsp. dill

Directions:

Firstly this dish will amaze you with its view, and then you will be surprised by its delicious taste. Take the bowl put oatmeal flour in it together. Add dill and oregano. Stir it. Take the bowl and pour warm water into it. Add baking soda and stir it till baking soda is dissolved. Combine oatmeal flour with liquid and knead the dough. Put it in the fridge. Meanwhile, chop the spinach and combine it with oatmeal. Take the tray and spray it with olive oil. Then take the dough and grate dough on it. Add spinach mass and stir it with the help of hands very gently. Preheat the air fryer and set at 180 C / 360 degrees F and transfer the tray with the mixture in it. Close the lid and then cook it for 15 minutes. Serve it immediately! Enjoy!

Nutrition:

Caloric content 319 kcal

Proteins 11.7 grams

Fats 6.3 grams

Carbohydrates 55.6 grams

Baked Veggie Salad

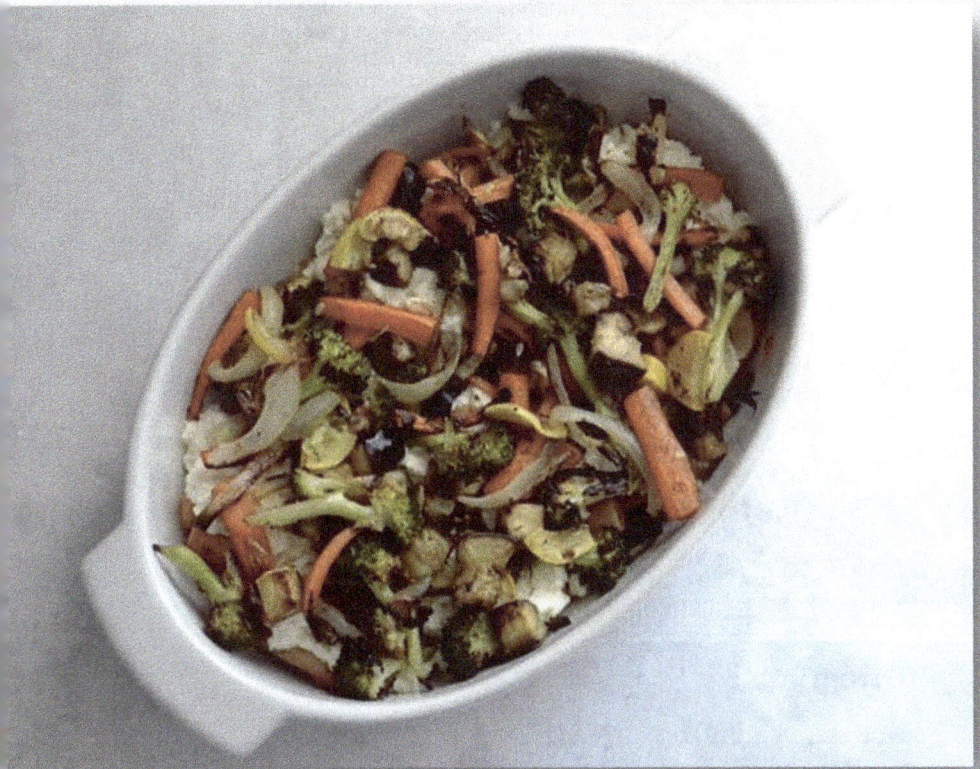

Preparation time: 10 minutes

Cooking time: 20 minutes

Servings: 4

Ingredients:

- Two red sweet peppers
- One sweet green pepper
- One red onion
- 100 g / 0.22 lbs. tofu
- Two tsp. lemon juice
- 50 g / 0.2 cup soy sauce
- One red apple
- 100 g / 0.4 cup water
- 200 g / 0.44 lbs. tomatoes
- 50 g / 1.76 oz. chopped chives
- 50 g / 0.2 cup soy milk
- 10 g / 0.35 oz. garlic
- One tsp. rice flour
- 50 g / 1.76 oz. quinoa

Directions:

Get the seeds from the sweet peppers and chop the pepper. Put it in the big bowl and sprinkle the vegetables with chopped chives and soy sauce. Stir it. Then chop the tomatoes and apples. Peel the onion and chop it too. All the vegetables should be chopped at the same size. Add them to the bowl with pepper mixture and stir it. Add rice flour, quinoa, and garlic. Stir the mass. Chop the tofu roughly and add it to the bowl too. Preheat the air fryer to 200 C / 390 F. Then pour soy milk into it and transfer the vegetable mixture to the air fryer. Cover with the lid and cook it for 10 minutes, not more. Open the lid and remove the salad from it. Sprinkle the salad with lemon juice and serve it immediately. Enjoy!

Tips: do not cook the salad for more than 10 minutes. Otherwise, the vegetables become soft and not delicious.

Nutrition:

Caloric content 159 kcal

Proteins 7.4 grams

Fats 2.6 grams

Carbohydrates 28.4 grams

Fragrant Quinoa

Preparation time: 10 minutes

Cooking time: 30 minutes

Servings: 4

Ingredients:

- 200 g / 0.44 lbs. quinoa
- 300 g / 1.2 cup vegetable stock
- One tsp. chilli pepper
- One tsp. rosemary
- One tsp. basil
- One tsp. turmeric
- One tsp. cilantro
- 100 g / 0.4 cup spinach
- 10 g / 0.35 oz. fresh mint
- 200 g / 0.44 lbs. tomatoes
- One red sweet pepper
- One tsp. black pepper

Directions:

Take the small bowl and combine chilli pepper, rosemary, basil, turmeric, cilantro, and spinach. Stir the mixture very carefully. Then remove the seeds from the sweet pepper and chop it.

Sprinkle the chopped peppers with the black pepper and stir it gently. Chop the tomatoes and mint. Take the big bowl and transfer all Ingredients to sprinkle the mass with the spice mixture then and stir it carefully. Leave it. Meanwhile, preheat the air fryer to 200 C / 390 F. Transfer the mixture to the air fryer and pour it with vegetable stock. Mix it using a wooden spoon. Close the lid and reduce the air fryer's heat to 180 C / 360 F. Cook the quinoa for 15 minutes or till it absorbs all water. Close the lid and remove the dish from the air fryer. Serve it immediately.

Tips: you can sprinkle the final dish with the mix of chopped dill and parsley.

Nutrition:

Caloric content 219 kcal

Proteins 9.0 grams

Fats 3.5 grams

Carbohydrates 38.7 grams

Delicious Festive Broccoli

Preparation time: 10 minutes

Cooking time: 20 minutes

Servings: 4

Ingredients:

- 400 g / 0.88 lbs. broccoli
- 100 g / 0.4 cup soy milk
- 100 g / 0.22 lbs. mushroom
- One yellow onion
- 10 g / 0.35 oz. almond flakes
- One tsp. white pepper
- 100 g / 0.22 lbs. grated tofu
- 30 g / 1 oz. chopped dill

Directions:

Take only fresh broccoli for this dish. Make the florets from the broccoli and sprinkle them with white pepper. Then take the big bowl and combine almond flakes and chopped dill in it. Add soy milk and stir the mass very gently. Then chop the tofu cheese and slice the mushrooms. Peel the onion and then chop it into tiny pieces. Combine chopped Ingredients and stir it. Preheat the air fryer to 190 C / 380 F and put the broccoli florets in it. Then pour it with liquid mass and add chopped vegetable mass.

Stir it with the help of the wooden or plastic spoon and close the lid. Cook it for 15 minutes. Remove the air fryer's dish and serve it immediately: firstly, put the broccoli on the plate, then pour it into a liquid mixture. Enjoy!

Nutrition:

Caloric content 116 kcal

Proteins 8.8 grams

Fats 3.5 grams

Carbohydrates 17.1 grams

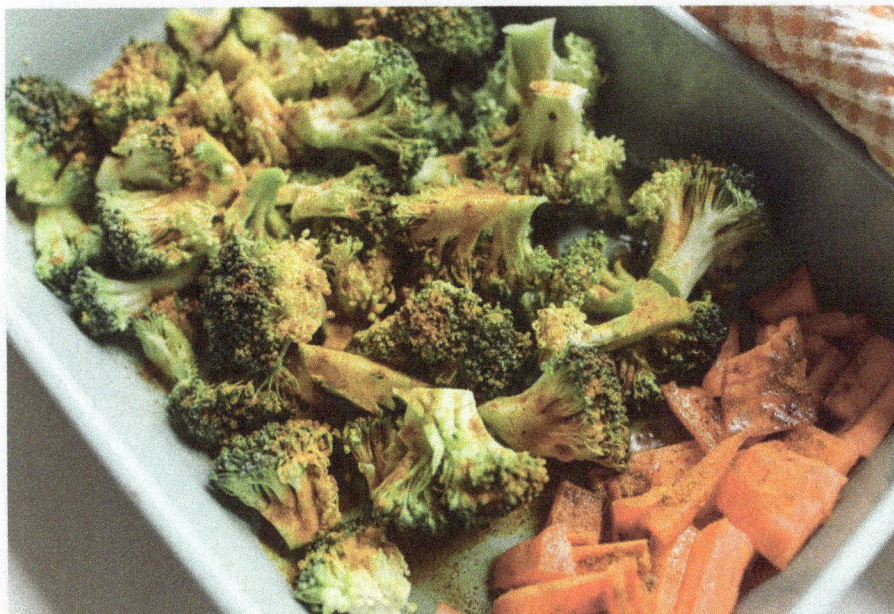

Baked Eggplant's Halves

Preparation time: 10 minutes

Cooking time: 30 minutes

Servings: 4

Ingredients:

- Four eggplants
- Two yellow onions
- 100 g / 0.4 cup soy milk
- One carrot
- 200 g / 0.44 lbs. tofu
- One tsp. olive oi l
- 100 g / 0.22 lbs. soy cheese
- One tsp. black pepper
- One tsp. basil
- One tsp. oregano
- 50 g / 1.76 oz. parsley
- 50 g / 0.2 cup water
- One tsp. salt

Directions:

Wash the eggplants and cut them into two parts. Then rub it with salt and leave it. Meanwhile, peel the yellow onions and chop them. Peel the carrot and grate it. Combine chopped the onion and grated carrot together. Sprinkle it with black pepper, basil, oregano and stir it carefully. Take the eggplants and remove the meat from them. Chop the meat and combine it with carrot and onion. Stir it. Chop the parsley and then put into the mixture too. Stir it again. Grate the tofu cheese. Preheat the air fryer to 190 C / 380 F. Pour the soy milk and water into the air fryer and stir it with the help of a wooden spoon. Fill the eggplants with the vegetable mass and sprinkle each half with grated tofu cheese. Transfer all eggplant's halves to the air fryer and close the lid. Cook it for 20 minutes. Then remove the dish from the air fryer and chill it a little. Enjoy!

Nutrition:

Caloric content 248 kcal

Proteins 12.0 grams

Fats 6.2 grams

Carbohydrates 43.2 grams

Super Vegetable Burger

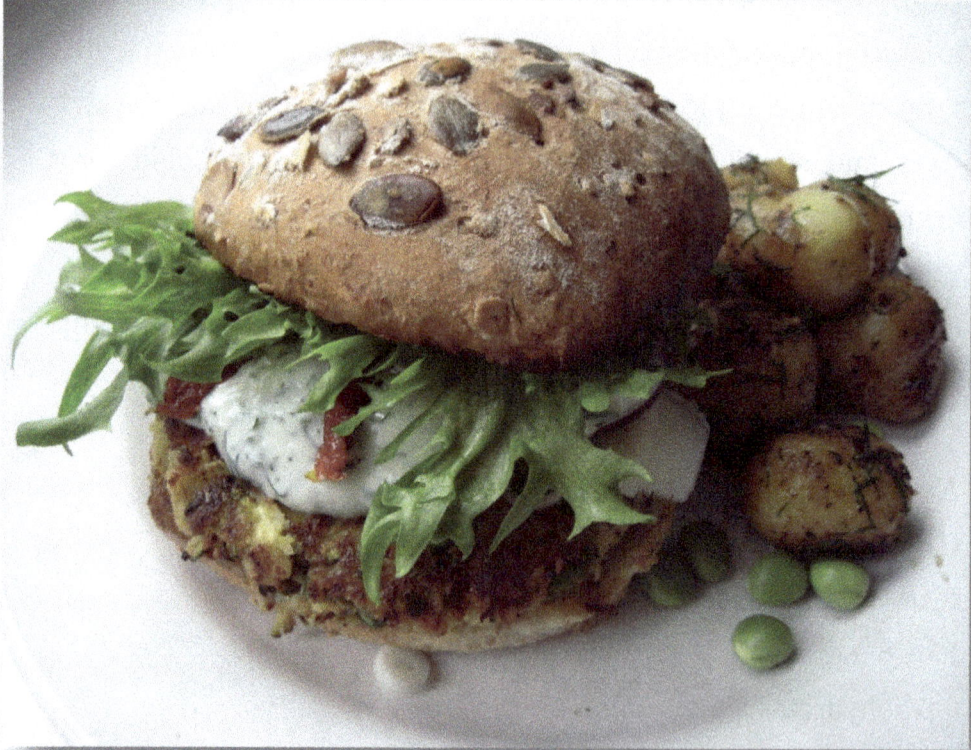

Preparation time: 10 minutes

Cooking time: 15 minutes

Servings: 4

Ingredients:

- 1/2-pound (227 g) cauliflower, steamed and diced, rinsed and drained
- Two tsp. coconut oil, melted
- Two tsp. minced garlic
- ¼ cup desiccated coconut
- ½ cup oats
- Three tbsp. flour
- One tbsp. flaxseeds plus three tbsp. water divided
- One tsp. thyme
- Two tsp. parsley
- Two tsp. chives
- Salt and ground black pepper, to taste
- 1 cup bread crumbs

Directions

Preheat and set the temperature at 390 F (199 C)

Combine the cauliflower with all the Ingredients, except for the bread crumbs, incorporating everything well

Using the hands, shape eight equal-sized amounts of the mixture into burger patties. Coat the patties in bread crumbs before putting them in the air fryer basket in a single layer

Place the basket of air fryers on the baking pan and move into position 2 of the rack. Select Air fry and set time to 12 minutes, or until crispy

Serve hot

Nutrition:

Energy (calories): 117 kcal

Protein: 4.97 g

Fat: 3.65 g

Carbohydrates: 21.58 g

Sweet Potatoes with Zucchini

Preparation time: 20 minutes

Cooking time: 20 minutes

Servings: 4

Ingredients:

- Two large-sized sweet potatoes, peeled and quartered
- One medium zucchini, sliced
- 1 Serrano pepper, deseeded and thinly sliced
- One bell pepper, deseeded and thinly sliced
- 1 to 2 carrots cut into matchsticks
- ¼ cup olive oil
- 1 ½ tbsp. maple syrup
- ½ tsp. porcini powder
- ½ tsp. fennel seeds
- One tbsp. garlic powder
- ½ tsp. fine sea salt
- ¼ tsp. ground black pepper
- Tomato ketchup, for serving

Directions:

Preheat the air fryer oven set at 350 F (177 C) degrees .

Put the sweet potatoes, zucchini, peppers, and carrot into the air fryer basket. Coat with a drizzling of olive oil

Place the air fryer basket on the baking pan and move into rack position2, pick the air fryer and set the time for 15 minutes.

In the meantime, prepare the sauce by vigorously combining the other Ingredients, except for tomato ketchup, with a whisk

Lightly grease a baking dish

Transfer the cooked vegetable to the baking dish, pour over the sauce and coat the vegetable well

Set the temperature at 390 F (199 C) and air fry the vegetable for an additional 5 minutes

Serve warm with a side of ketchup

Nutrition:

Energy (calories): 247 kcal

Protein: 3.05 g

Fat: 13.84 g

Carbohydrates: 29.74 g

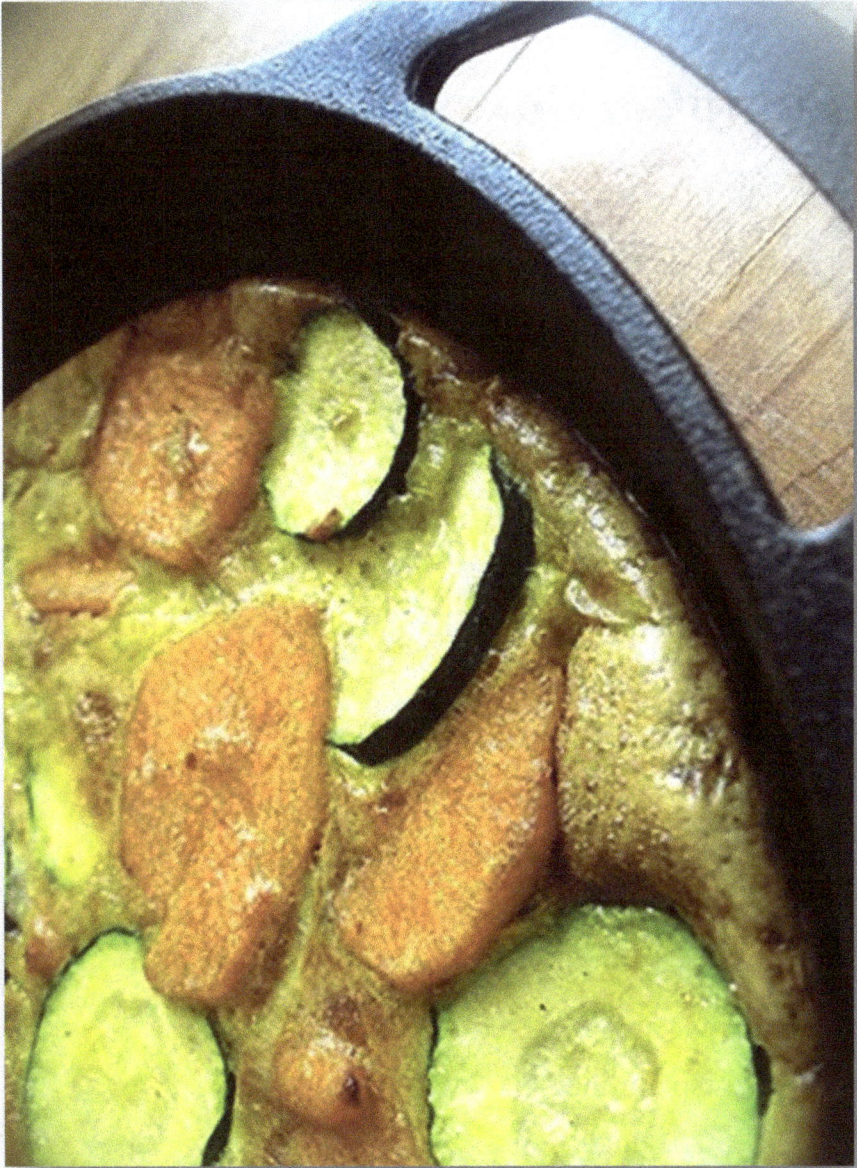

Vegan Fruits

Pumpkin Bars

Preparation time: 10 minutes
Cooking time: 25 minutes
Servings: 6

Ingredients:
- ¼ cup almond butter
- 1 tbsp. unsweetened almond milk
- ½ cup coconut flour
- ¾ tsp. baking soda
- ½ cup dark sugar-free chocolate chips, divided
- 1 cup canned sugar-free pumpkin puree
- ¼ cup swerve
- 1 tsp. cinnamon
- 1 tsp. vanilla extract
- ¼ tsp. nutmeg
- ½ tsp. ginger
- 1/8 tsp. salt
- 1/8 tsp. ground cloves

Directions:

Preheat the Air fryer to 360 o F and layer a baking pan with wax paper.

Mix pumpkin puree, swerve, vanilla extract, milk, and butter in a bowl.

Combine coconut flour, spices, salt, and baking soda in another bowl.

Put together the two mixtures and mix well until smooth.

Add about 1/3 cup of the sugar-free chocolate chips and transfer this mixture into the baking pan.

Transfer into the Air fryer basket and cook for about 25 minutes.

Microwave sugar-free chocolate bits on low heat and dish out the baked cake from the pan.

Top with melted chocolate and slice to serve.

Nutrition:

Calories: 249

Fat: 11.9g

Carbohydrates: 1.8g

Sugar: 0.3g

Protein: 5g

Sodium: 79mg

Strawberry Cobbler Recipe

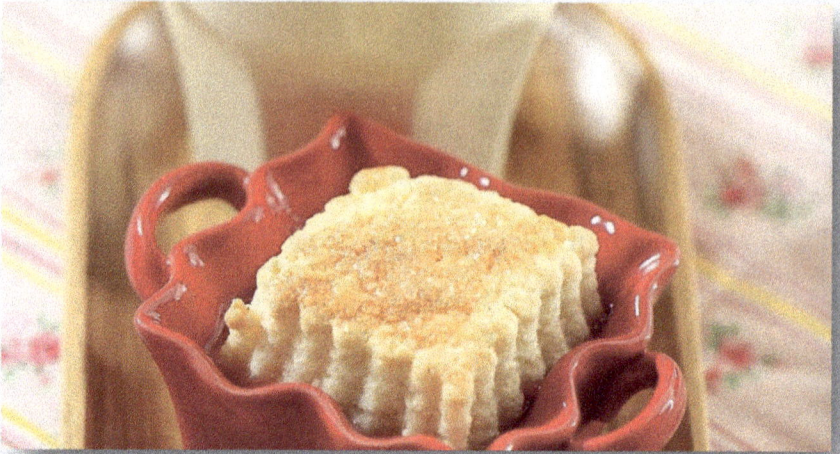

Preparation time: 10 minutes

Cooking time: 25 minutes

Servings: 6

Ingredients:

- 3/4 cup sugar
- 6 cups strawberries; halved
- 1/2 cup flour
- 1/8 tsp. baking powder
- 1/2 cup water

- 3 ½ tbsp. olive oil
- 1 tbsp. lemon juice
- A pinch of baking soda
- Coconut oil

Directions:

In a bowl, mix strawberries with half of the sugar, sprinkle some flour, add lemon juice, whisk and pour into the baking dish that fits your air fryer and greased with Coconut oil.

In another bowl, mix flour with the rest of the sugar, baking powder and soda and stir well

Add the olive oil and then mix until the whole thing with your hands

Add 1/2 cup water and spread over strawberries

Introduce in the fryer at 355°F and bake for 25 minutes. Leave cobbler aside to cool down, slice and serve.

Nutrition:

Energy (calories): 203 kcal

Protein: 2.05 g

Fat: 8.42 g

Carbohydrates: 31.66 g

Cranberry Jam

Preparation time: 5 minutes

Cooking time: 20 minutes

Servings: 8

Preparation time: 25 minutes

Ingredients:

- 2 lbs. cranberries
- 4 oz. black currant
- 3 tbsp. water
- 2 lbs. sugar
- Zest of 1 lime

Directions:

In a pan that fits exactly on your air fryer, add all the Ingredients and stir.

Place the pan in the fryer and cook at 360°F for 20 minutes. Stir the jam well, divide into cups, refrigerate and serve cold

Nutrition:

Energy (calories): 513 kcal

Protein: 0.22 g

Fat: 0.18 g

Carbohydrates:131.11g

Apple-Toffee Upside-Down Cake

Preparation time: 5 minutes

Cooking time: 30 minutes

Servings: 9

Ingredients:
- ¼ cup almond butter
- ¼ cup sunflower oil
- ½ cup walnuts, chopped
- ¾ cup + 3 tbsp. coconut sugar
- ¾ cup of water
- 1 ½ tsp. mixed spice
- 1 cup plain flour
- 1 lemon, zest
- 1 tsp. baking soda
- 1 tsp. vinegar
- 3 baking apples, cored and sliced

Directions:

Preheat the air fryer to 390OF.

In a skillet, melt the almond butter and three tbsp. of sugar.

Pour the mixture over a baking dish that will fit in the air fryer.

Arrange the slices of apples on top. Set aside.

In a mixing bowl, combine flour, ¾ cup sugar, and baking soda. Add the mixed spice.

In another bowl, mix the sunflower oil, water, vinegar, and lemon zest. Stir in the chopped walnuts.

Combine the wet Ingredients to the dry Ingredients until well combined.

Pour over the tin with apple slices.

Bake and cook for about 30 minutes or until a toothpick inserted comes out clean.

Nutrition:

Calories: 335

Carbohydrates: 39.6g

Protein: 3.8g

Fat: 17.9g

Yummy Banana Cookies

Preparation time: 5 minutes

Cooking time: 20 minutes

Servings: 6

Ingredients:

- 1 cup dates, pitted and chopped
- 1 tsp. vanilla
- 1/3 cup vegetable oil
- cups rolled oats
- ripe bananas

Directions:

Preheat the air fryer to 350oF.

In a prepared bowl, mash the bananas and add in the rest of the Ingredients.

Let it rest inside the fridge for 10 minutes.

Drop a tsp. on cut parchment paper.

Place the cookies on parchment paper inside the air fryer basket. Make sure that the cookies do not overlap. Cook for about 20 minutes or until the edges are crispy.

Serve with almond milk.

Nutrition:

Calories: 382

Carbohydrates: 50.14g

Protein: 6.54g

Fat: 17.2g

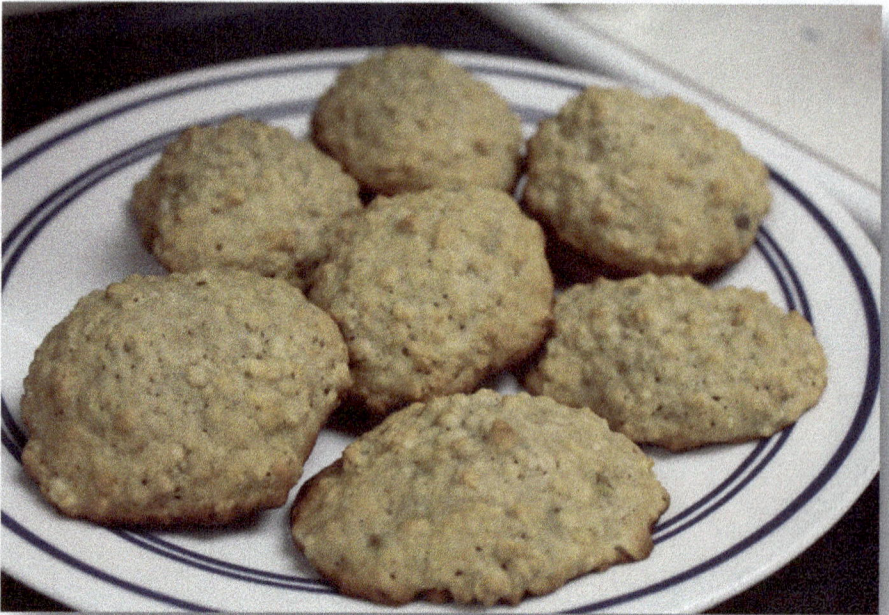

Raspberry Wontons

Preparation time: 20 minutes
Cooking time: 16 minutes
Servings: 12

Ingredients:

- For Wonton Wrappers:
- ½ cup Coconut sugar
- 18 ounces vegan cheese, softened
- 1 tsp. vanilla extract
- 1 package of vegan wonton wrappers
- For Raspberry Syrup:
- ¼ cup of water
- ¼ cup sugar
- 1: 12-ounce package frozen raspberries
- 1 tsp. vanilla extract

Directions:

For wrappers: in a bowl, add the sugar, vegan cheese, and vanilla extract and whisk until smooth.

Place a wonton wrapper onto a smooth surface.

Place one tbsp. of vegan cheese mixture in the center of each wrapper.

With wet fingers, fold wrappers around the filling and pinch the edges to seal.

Set the air fryer's temperature to 350 degrees F. Lightly grease an air fryer basket.

Arrange wonton wrappers into the prepared air fryer basket in 2 batches.

Air fry for about 8 minutes.

Meanwhile, for the syrup: in a medium skillet, add water, sugar, raspberries, and vanilla extract over medium heat and cook for about 5 minutes, stirring continuously.

Remove from the heat and set aside to cool slightly.

Transfer the mixture into the food processor and blend until smooth.

Remove the wontons from the air fryer and transfer them onto a platter.

Serve the wontons with a topping of raspberry syrup.

Nutrition:

Calories: 325

Carbohydrate: 39.6g

Protein: 7.1g

Fat: 15.5g

Sugar: 15.4g

Sodium: 343mg

Fruit Sandwich

Preparation time: 10 minutes
Cooking time: 10minutes
Servings: 2

Ingredients:

- 2 slices of sandwich
- Green apple
- Banana
- Maple syrup

Directions:

Slicing the apple and the banana finely

Fry the apple (to caramelize) and slices of bread for 6 minutes in Air Fryer at 160°F.

To Plate: Serve up the sandwich with banana slices and caramelized apple. Bathe with Maple syrup.

Nutrition:

Energy (calories): 47 kcal

Protein: 0.24 g

Fat: 0.15 g

Carbohydrates: 12.57 g

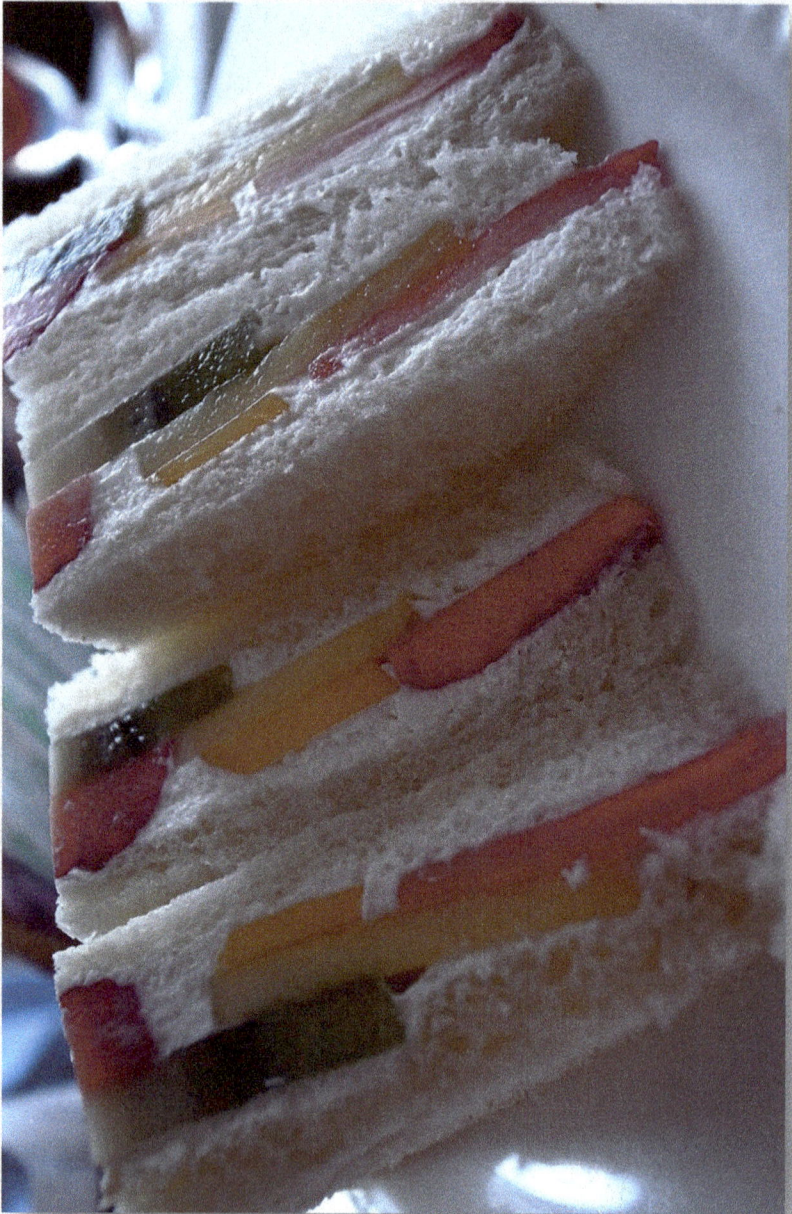

Candy Apple

Preparation time: 5 minutes

Cooking time: 10 minutes

Servings: 2

Ingredients:

- Apple
- Salt.
- Brown sugar.
- Apple vinegar

Directions:

Peel the apple, remove the seed and cut into segments.

Season with the other Ingredients, place them in a metal mould varnished with a little oil and bring to the Air Fryer for 5 minutes at 180 °C. It is stirred so that it cooks evenly.

Nutrition:

Energy (calories): 47 kcal

Protein: 0.24 g

Fat: 0.15 g

Carbohydrates: 12.57 g

Vegan Dessert

Pumpkin Pie

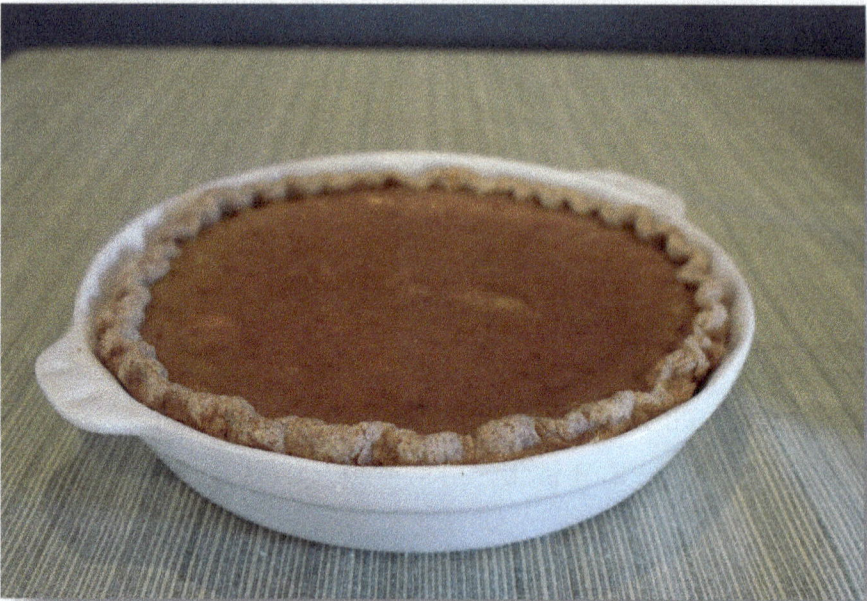

Preparation time: 10 minutes

Cooking time: 15 minutes

Servings: 9

Ingredients:

- One tbsp. sugar
- Two tbsp. flour
- One tbsp. vegan butte r
- Two tbsp. water
- For the pumpkin pie filling:
- 3.5 ounces pumpkin flesh, chopped
- One tsp. mixed spice
- One tsp. nutmeg
- 3 ounces of water
- ¼ cup vegan Buttermilk
- One tbsp. sugar

Directions:

Put 3 ounces water in a pot, bring to a boil over medium-high heat, add pumpkin, vegan buttermilk, one tbsp. sugar, spice and nutmeg, stir, boil for 20 minutes, take off the heat and blend using an immersion blender.

In a bowl, mix flour with butter, one tbsp. sugar and two tbsp. water and knead your dough well.

Grease a pie pan that fits your air fryer with vegan butter, press dough into the pan, fill with pumpkin pie filling, place in your air fryer's basket and cook at 360 degrees F for 15 minutes.

Slice and serve warm.

Enjoy!

Nutrition:

Calories 200

Fat 5

Fiber 2

Carbs 5

Protein 6

Coconut Pineapples & Vegan Yoghurt Dip

Preparation time: 15 minutes
Cooking time: 10 minutes
Servings: 4

Ingredients:

- 2 ounces of dried coconut flakes
- One sprig of mint, finely chopped
- ½ medium size pineapples
- 8 ounces of vegan yogurt

Directions:

Heat the Air Fryer to 390°F.

Slice the pineapple into chips (sticks) and dip them into the diced coconut to allow the coconut to stick to them.

Place the sticks in the fryer basket and cook for about 10 minutes.

Stir the mint leaves into the vegan yogurt. Serve with pineapple sticks.

Nutrition:

Energy (calories): 118 kcal

Protein: 15.93 g

Fat: 4.59 g

Carbohydrates: 2.57 g

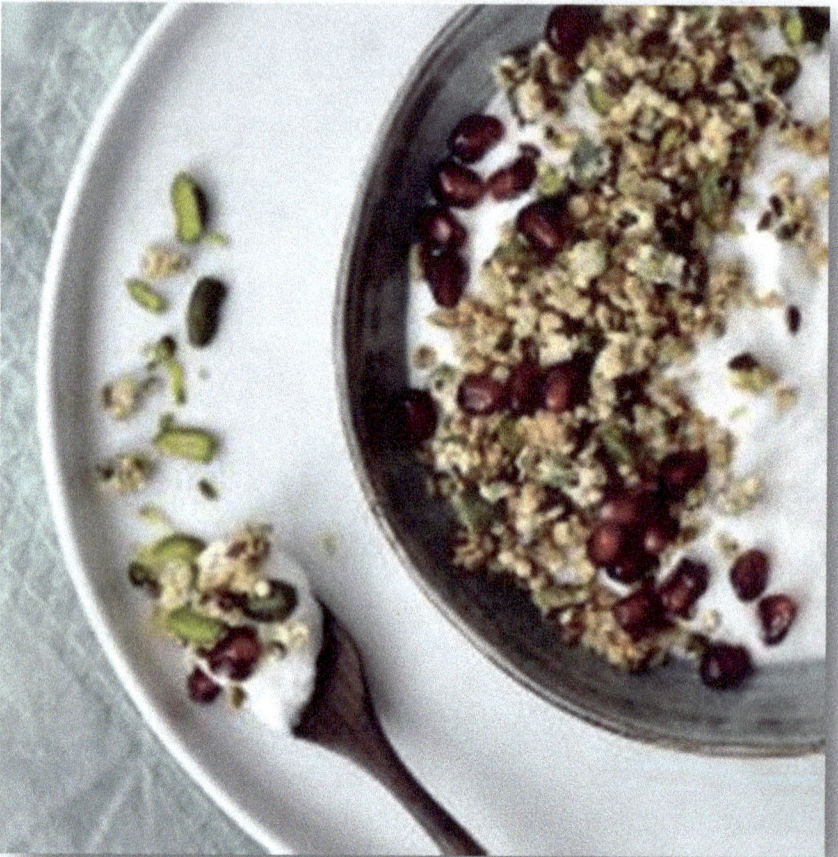

Stuffed Apple Bake

Preparation time: 5 minutes

Cooking time: 10 minutes

Servings: 4

Ingredients:

- Four medium-sized apples, cored
- Six tsp. of sugar
- Four tbsp. of breadcrumbs
- Two tbsp. of vegan butter
- One tsp. of mixed spice
- 1½ ounce of mixed seeds Zest of
- One lemon

Directions:

Score the apples' skin with a knife around the circumference to prevent them from dividing during baking.

Mix the sugar, breadcrumbs, vegan butter, zest, spice and mixed seeds in a bowl and stuff the apples with the mixture.

Heat the Air Fryer at 356°F and bake the stuffed apples for 10 minutes.

Nutrition:

Energy (calories): 117 kcal

Protein: 2.98 g

Fat: 8.4 g

Carbohydrates: 9.68 g

Berry and Apricot Crumble

Preparation time: 10 minutes
Cooking time: 20 minutes
Servings: 6

Ingredients:

- 2½ ounces of vegan butter
- 2¼ cups of apricot
- ½ pound of flour
- Eight tbsp. of sugar
- Six tsp. of lemon juice
- 5½ ounces fresh blackberries Salt to tast e

Directions:

Cut the apricots into two and take out the stone, then cut into cubes.

Put them in a bowl and add two tbsp. of sugar, the blackberries and lemon juice and stir. Pour and spread the mixture evenly in an oven dish.

Place the flour in a prepared bowl and add six tbsp. of sugar, the vegan butter, salt, and a little water and mix thoroughly. Rub the mixture with your fingertips until crumbly.

Heat your Air Fryer to 390°F.

Spread the mixture on the fruits and press down lightly.
Put into the Air Fryer basket and bake for 20 minutes until the crumble appears golden.

Nutrition:

Energy (calories): 369 kcal

Protein: 6 g

Fat: 10.24 g

Carbohydrates: 66.78 g

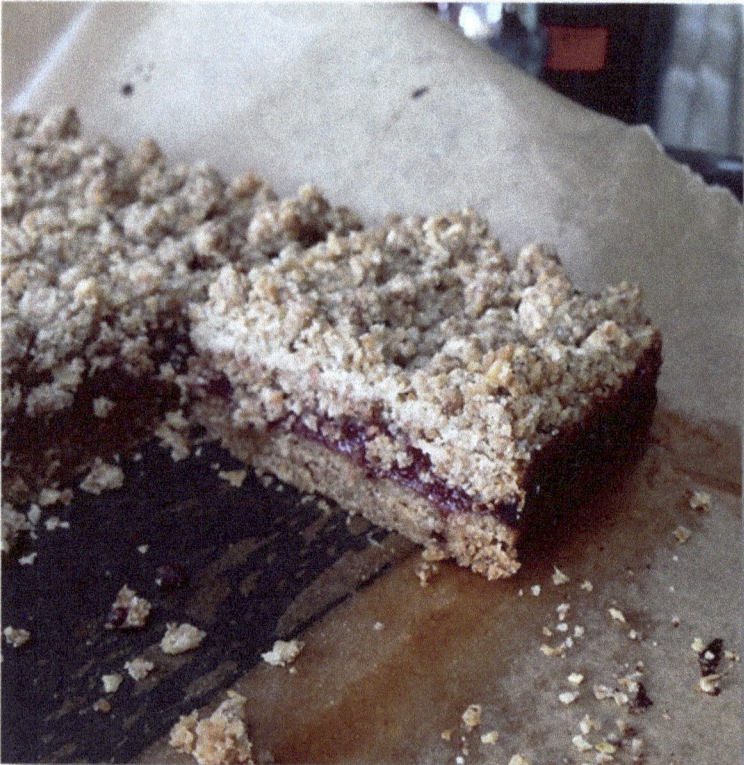

Sponge Cake

Preparation time: 10 minutes

Cooking time: 20 minutes

Servings: 12

Ingredients:

- 3 cups flour
- Three tsp. baking powder
- ½ cup cornstarch
- One tsp. baking soda
- 1 cup olive oil
- One and ½ cup of almond milk
- 1 and 2/3 cup sugar
- 2 cups of water
- ¼ cup lemon juice
- 2 tsp. vanilla extract

Directions:

In a bowl, mix flour with cornstarch, baking powder, baking soda and sugar and whisk well.

In another bowl, mix oil with almond milk, water, vanilla and lemon juice and whisk.

Combine the two mixtures, stir, pour in a greased baking dish that fits your air fryer, introduce in the fryer and cook at 350 degrees F for 20 minutes.

Leave the cake to cool down, cut and serve.

Enjoy!

Nutrition:

Energy (calories): 334 kcal

Protein: 3.32 g

Fat: 18.45 g

Carbohydrates: 38.6 g

Blueberry Pudding

Preparation time: 10 minutes

Cooking time: 25 minutes

Servings: 6

Ingredients:

- 2 cups flour
- 2 cups rolled oats
- 8 cups blueberries
- One stick vegan butter, melted
- 1 cup walnuts, chopped
- 3 tbsp. maple syrup
- 2 tbsp. rosemary, chopped

Directions:

Spread blueberries in a greased baking pan and leave them aside.

In your food processor, mix rolled oats with the flour, walnuts, vegan butter, maple syrup and rosemary, blend well, layer this over blueberries, introduce everything in your air fryer and cook at 350 degrees for 25 minutes.

Leave dessert to cool down, cut and serve.

Enjoy!

Nutrition:

Calories 150

Fat 3g

Fibre 2g

Carbs 7g

Protein 4g

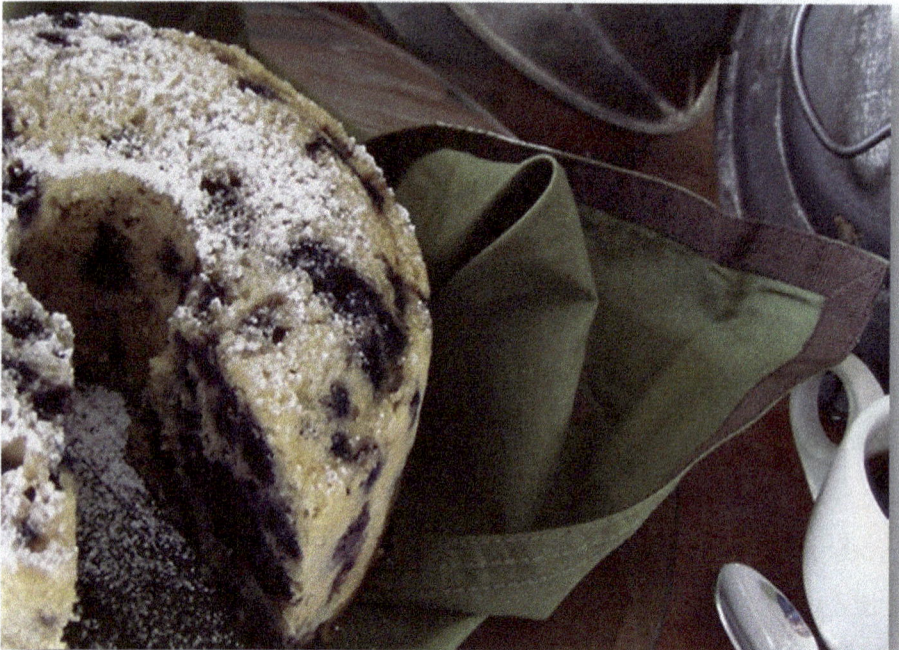

Cocoa and Almond Bars

Preparation time: 30 minutes
Cooking time: 4 minutes
Servings: 6

Ingredients:

- ¼ cup cocoa nibs
- 1 cup almonds, soaked and drained
- 2 tbsps. cocoa powder
- ¼ cup hemp seeds
- ¼ cup goji berries
- ¼ cup coconut, shredded
- Eight dates, pitted and soake d

Directions:

Put almonds in your food processor, blend, add hemp seeds, cocoa nibs, cocoa powder, goji, coconut and blend very well.

Add dates, blend well again, spread on a lined baking sheet that fits your air fryer and cooks at 320 degrees F for 4 minutes.

Cut into equal parts and keep in the fridge for 30 minutes before serving.

Enjoy!

Nutrition:

Calories 140

Fat 6g

Fibre 3g

Carbs 7g

Protein 1g

Chocolate and Pomegranate Bars

Preparation time: 120 minutes

Cooking time: 10 minutes

Servings: 6

Ingredients:

- ½ cup almond milk
- 1 tsp. vanilla extract
- One and ½ cups dark chocolate, chopped
- ½ cup almonds, chopped
- ½ cup pomegranate seeds

Directions:

Heat a pan with the almond milk over medium-low heat, add chocolate, stir for 5 minutes, take off heat add vanilla extract, half of the pomegranate seeds and half of the nuts and stir.

Pour this into a lined baking pan, spread, sprinkle a pinch of salt, the rest of the pomegranate arils and nuts, introduce in your air fryer and cook at 300 degrees F for 4 minutes.

Keep in the fridge for 2 hours before serving.

Enjoy!

Nutrition:

Calories 68

Fat 1g

Fibre 4g

Carbs 6g

Protein 1g

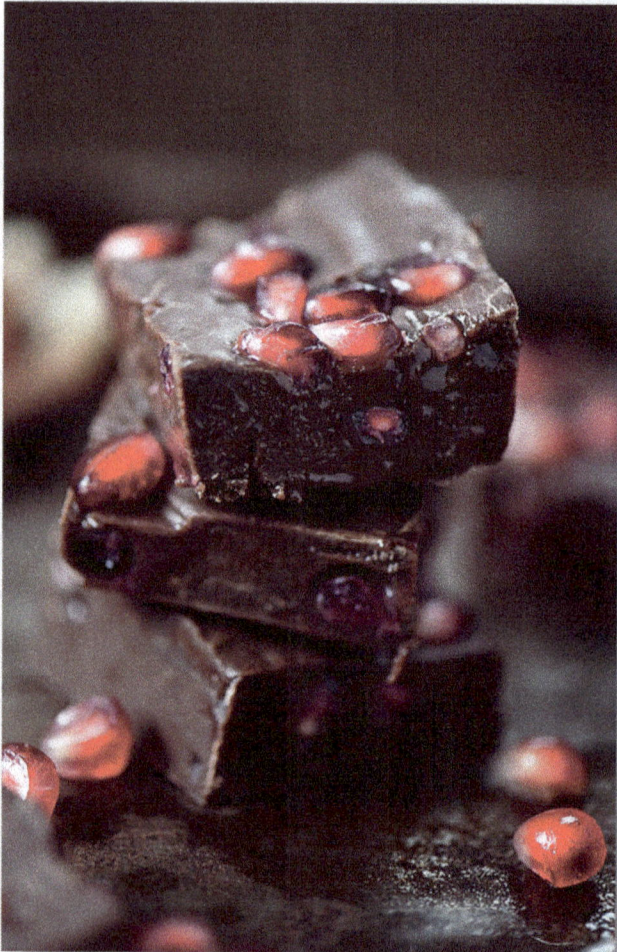

Vegan Snacks

Rice Balls

Preparation time: 10 minutes

Cooking time: 35 minutes

Servings: 6

Ingredients:

- One small yellow onion, chopped
- 1 cup Arborio rice
- 1 tbsp. olive oil
- 1 cup veggie stock
- Salt and black pepper to the taste
- 2 ounces tofu, cubed
- ¼ cup sun-dried tomatoes, chopped
- One and ½ cups vegan breadcrumbs
- A drizzle of olive oil
- Marinara sauce for serving

Directions:

Heat a pan with 1 tbsp. oil over medium heat, add onion, stir and cook for 5 minutes.

Add rice, stock, salt and pepper, stir, and cook on low heat for 20 minutes, spread on a baking sheet and leave aside to cool down.

Transfer rice to a bowl, add tomatoes and half of the breadcrumbs and stir well.

Shape 12 balls, press a hole in each ball, stuff with tofu cubes, and mould them again.

Dredge them in the rest of the breadcrumbs, arrange all balls in your air fryer, drizzle the oil over them and cook at 380 degrees F for 10 minutes.

Flip them and cook for 5 minutes more.

Arrange them on a plate and then serve them as a snack.

Enjoy!

Nutrition:

Calories 137

Fat 12g

Fiber 1g

Carbs 7g

Protein 5g

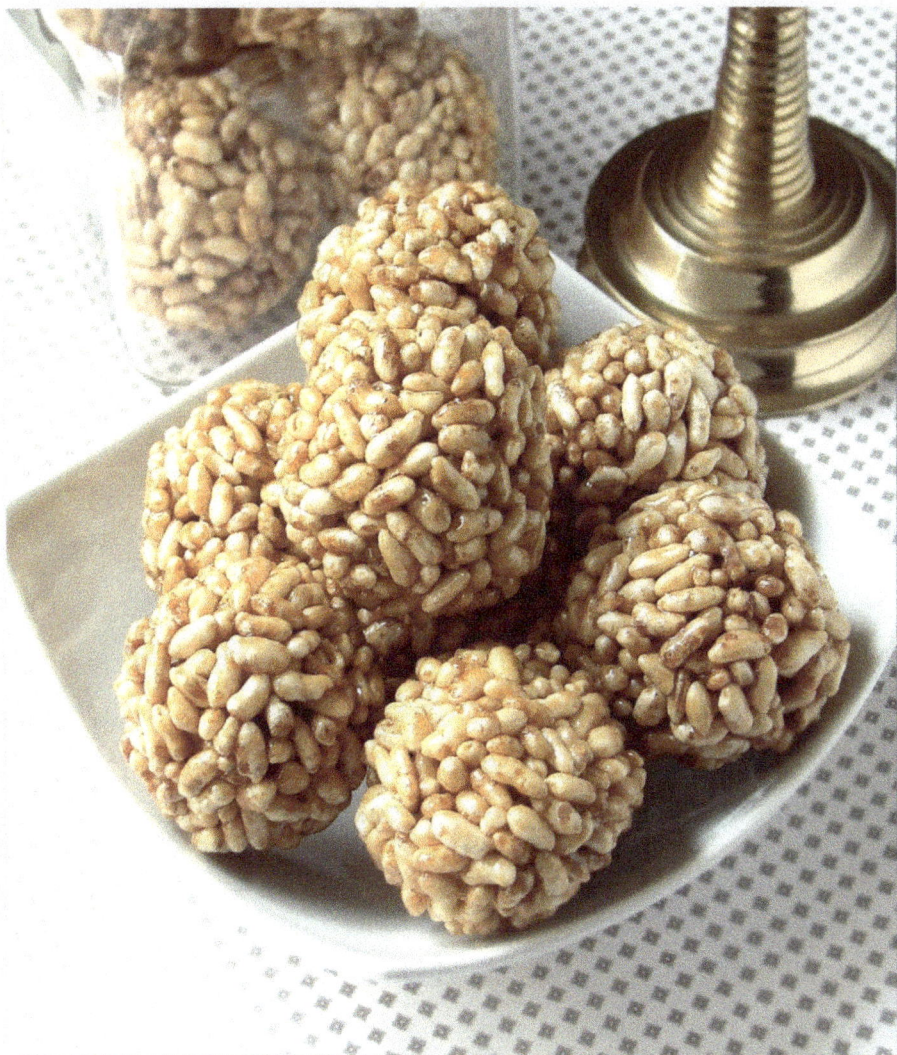

Tofu Snack

Preparation time: 30 minutes

Cooking time: 20 minutes

Servings: 4

Ingredients:

- 12 ounces firm tofu, cubed
- 1 tsp. sweet paprika
- 1 tsp. sesame oil
- 1 tbsp. coriander, chopped
- 2 tbsp. coconut aminos

Directions:

In a bowl, mix paprika with the oil, coriander and amino, whisk well, add tofu pieces, toss to coat and leave aside for 30 minutes.

Transfer tofu cubes to your air fryer's basket and cook at 350 degrees F for 20 minutes, shaking halfway.

Transfer them to a bowl and serve as a snack.

Enjoy!

Nutrition:

Calories 90

Fat 2g

Fiber 1g

Carbs 6g

Protein 1g

Apple Chips

Preparation time: 10 minutes

Cooking time: 15 minutes

Servings: 2

Ingredients:

- One apple, cored and thinly sliced
- ½ tsp. cinnamon powder
- 1 tbsp. stevia

Directions:

Arrange apple slices in your air fryer's basket, add stevia and cinnamon, toss and cook at 390 degrees F for 10 minutes, turning them halfway.

Transfer to a bowl and serve as a snack.

Enjoy!

Nutrition:

Calories 90

Fat 0g

Fiber 4g

Carbs 12g

Protein 4 g

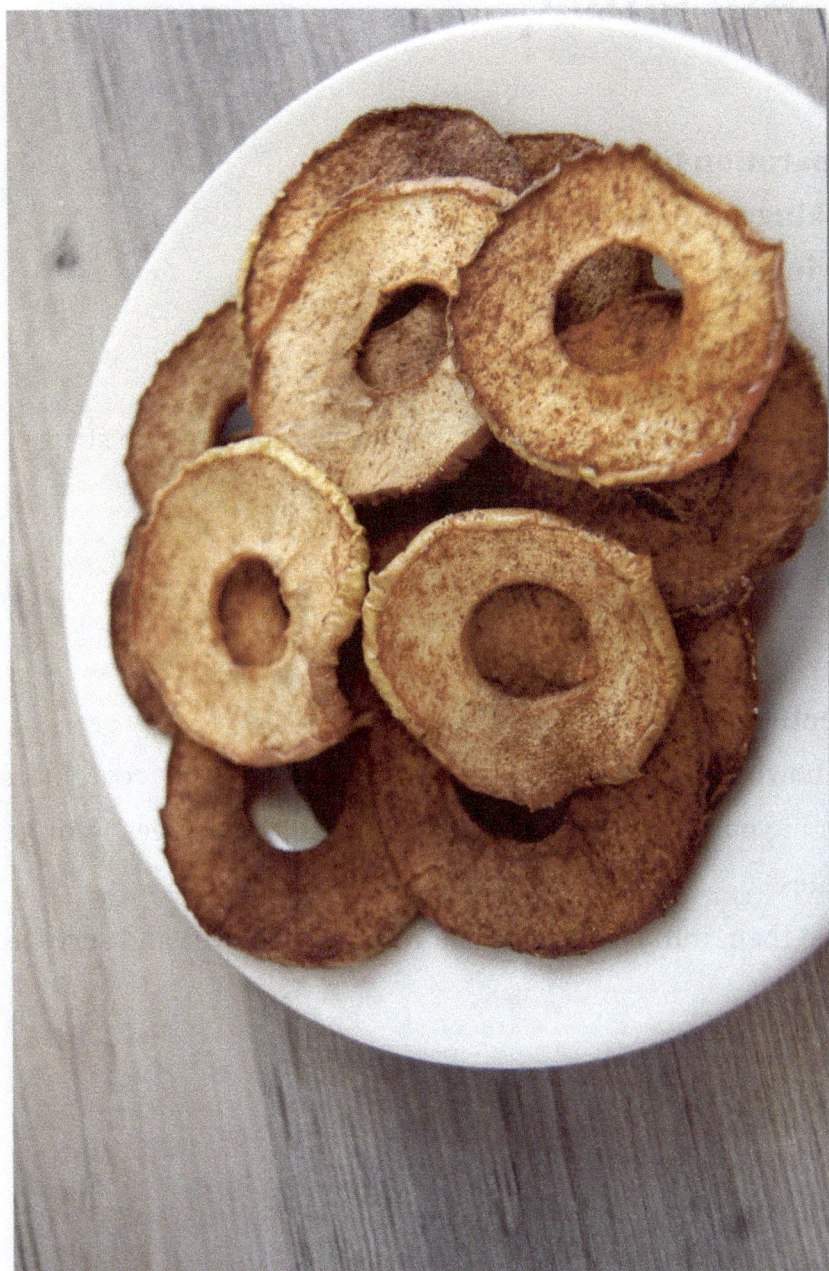

Potato Chips

Preparation time: 30 minutes
Cooking time: 30 minutes
Servings: 4

Ingredients:

- Four potatoes, scrubbed, peeled and cut into thin strips
- A pinch of sea salt
- 1 tbsp. olive oil
- 2 tsp. rosemary, chopped

Directions:

In a bowl, mix potato chips with salt and oil, toss to coat, place them in your air fryer's basket and cook at 330 degrees F for 30 minutes.

Divide them into bowls, sprinkle rosemary all over and serve as a snack.

Enjoy!

Nutrition:

Calories 200

Fat 4g

Fiber 4g

Carbs 14g

Protein 5g

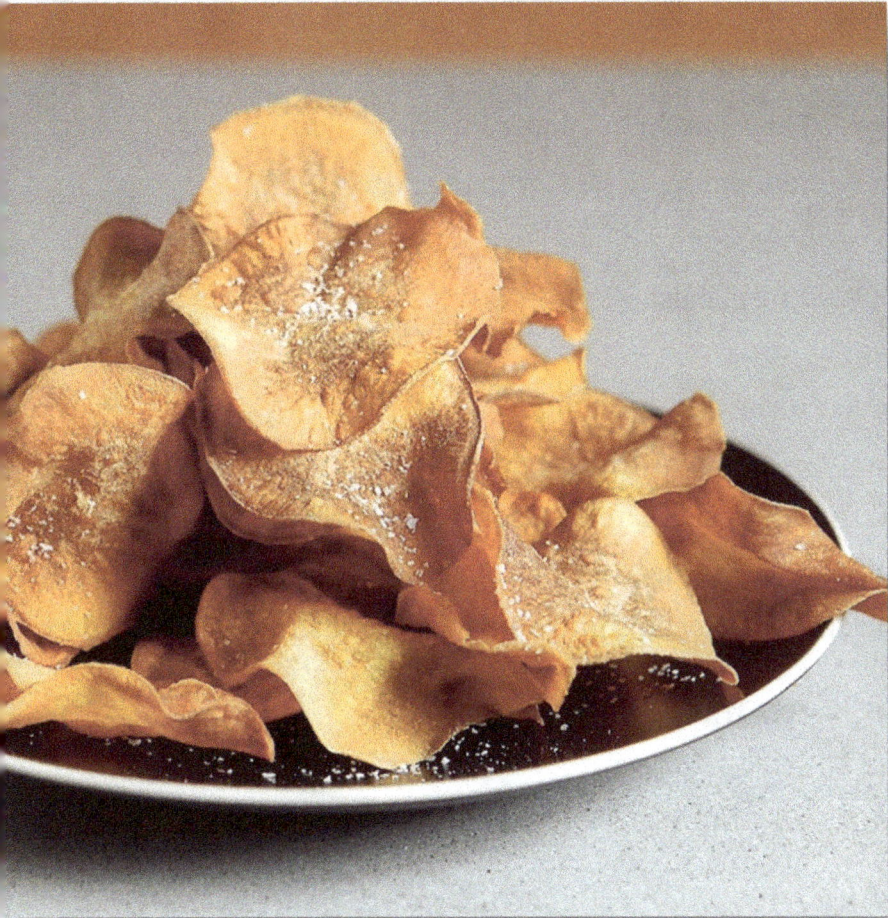

Easy Zucchini Chips

Preparation time: 10 minutes

Cooking time: 30 minutes

Servings: 6

Ingredients:

- Three zucchinis, thinly sliced
- Salt and black pepper to the taste
- 2 tbsp. olive oil
- 2 tbsp. balsamic vinegar

Directions:

In a bowl, mix oil with vinegar, salt and pepper and whisk well.
Add zucchini slices, toss to coat well, introduce in your air fryer
and cook at 350 degrees F for 30 minutes.
Divide zucchini chips into bowls and serve them cold as a snack.
Enjoy!

Nutrition:

Calories 100

Fat 3g

Fiber 2g

Carbs 6g

Protein 7g

Vegan Bread and Pizza

Mixed Bread Or Rolls Made From Rye And Wheat (Vegan)

Preparation time: 10 minutes

Cooking time: 40 minutes

Servings: 1bread

Ingredients:

- 150 g rye flour
- 150 g wheat flour
- 280 ml of lukewarm water
- ½ yeast cube
- 1 tbsp. salt

Directions:

Put salt, rye and wheat flour in a bowl and mix. Make a well in the middle and add the yeast cubes. Pour lukewarm water over and let it rest for 10 minutes so that the yeast dissolves. Then knead all the Ingredients into a dough and cover with a clean kitchen towel. Let it rest in a warm place for 30 minutes.

Now, shape a bread or four rolls out of the dough. Grease the baking pan of the air fryer, sprinkle with flour, alternatively line with baking paper. Now put the bread or rolls in the mould and bake at 200 ° C (rolls 25 minutes, bread for 35 minutes).

Nutrition:

Energy (calories): 357 kcal

Protein: 10.61 g

Fat: 1.25 g

Carbohydrates: 75.87 g

Spicy Sourdough Bread (Vegan)

Preparation time: 10 minutes

Cooking time: 40 minutes

Servings: 1bread

Ingredients:

- 500g flour
- 75 g ready-made sourdough
- ½ yeast cube
- 1 tbsp. salt
- 375 ml of water
- ½ tsp. rosemary
- ½ tsp. marjoram
- ½ tsp. tarragon

Directions:

Mix the flour with salt, rosemary, marjoram and tarragon. Crumble the yeast and dissolve in lukewarm water. Mix with the flour and herbs. Add the sourdough and knead everything into a dough. Cover with a clean kitchen towel and let rise for about an hour.

Grease the bread pan and then sprinkle with flour, or line with baking paper. Pour in the dough and let it rest for another 30 minutes. Now sprinkle the dough with a little flour and bake in the air fryer for 35 minutes at 200 ° C.

Nutrition:

Energy (calories): 1880 kcal

Protein: 54.06 g

Fat: 6.34 g

Carbohydrates: 391.03 g

Spelled Bread (Vegan)

Preparation time: 10 minutes

Cooking time: 45 minutes

Servings: 1bread

Ingredients:

- 500 g spelled flour
- 1 tbsp. salt
- One yeast cube
- 250 ml of lukewarm water
- One pinch of sugar
- 1 tsp. anise

Directions:

Put flour, salt and anise in a bowl and mix. Make a well in the middle and crumble the yeast into it. Pour a pinch of sugar over it. Cover the yeast and sugar with lukewarm water and let rest for 10 minutes so that the yeast dissolves.

Mix all Ingredients in the bowl and knead into a dough. Cover with a clean kitchen towel and let rise in a warm place for about 60 minutes.

Line the breadbasket of the air fryer with baking paper or grease and dust with flour. Put the dough in the breadbasket of the Airfryer and bake for 30-35 minutes at 200 ° C.

Nutrition:

Energy (calories): 1827 kcal

Protein: 52.02 g

Fat: 5.23 g

Carbohydrates: 382.6 g

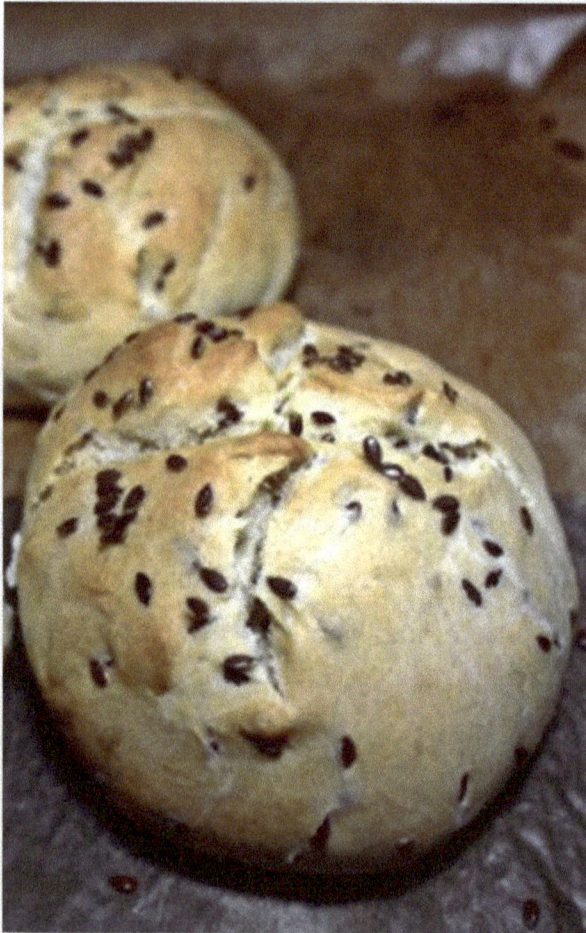

Vegan Cookies with Chocolate Sparks

Preparation time: 15 minutes
Cooking time: 15 minutes
Servings: 2

Ingredients:

- 2 ½ cups of whole wheat flour
- 1 cup brown sugar
- ½ tsp. baking soda
- ¼ tsp. salt
- ½ cup unsweetened non-dairy milk
- ¼ cup of coconut oil
- 2 flax eggs
- 1 tsp. vanilla extract
- ¾ cup vegan chocolate chips

Directions:

Preheat the air fryer to 350°F .

Mix all dry Ingredients in a prepared large bowl (the flour, sugar, baking soda, and salt).

Add the liquid Ingredients to the large bowl and stir until well combined.

Add the chocolate chips and stir until well combined. Let the dough rest in the fridge for 30 minutes to make it easier to handle.

Put one scoop of ice cream per cookie on a baking sheet lined with parchment paper and flatten them with your hands a little to shape them.

Bake for about 15 minutes or until they start to brown on the sides.

Nutrition:

Calories: 84.3

Carbohydrates: 11.8g

Fat: 2.7g

Protein: 2.1g

Sugar: 3.4g

Cholesterol: 0.5mg

Vegan Main Dishes

Carrot & Potato Mix

Preparation time: 10 minutes

Cooking time: 16 minutes

Servings: 6

Ingredients:

- Potatoes (2)
- Carrots (3 lb.)
- Yellow onion (1)
- Dried thyme (1 tsp.)
- Black pepper and salt (to your liking)
- Curry powder (2 tsp.)
- Coconut milk (3 tbsp.)
- Vegan cheese (3 tbsp.)
- Parsley (1 tbsp.)

Directions:

Cube/chop the parsley, carrots, and onions. Crumble the vegan cheese.

Warm the Air Fryer to reach 365° Fahrenheit.

Once it's heated, toss in the veggies, thyme, curry powder, salt, and pepper. Set the timer and air-fry for 16 minutes .

Stir in the milk and cheese.

Portion and serve.

Nutrition

Protein Count: 4 grams

Carbohydrates: 1 gram

Fat Content: 4 grams

Calorie: 241

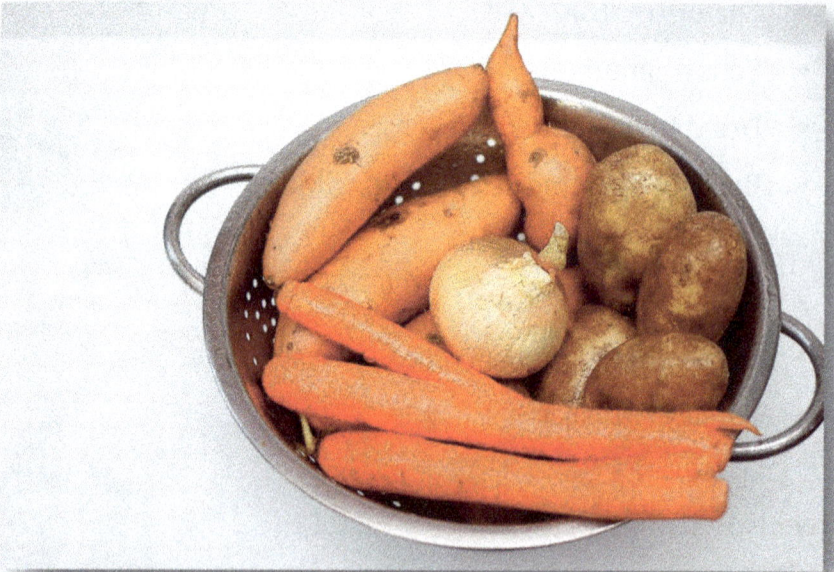

Eggplant Fries

"Ditch the traditional eggplants and fry them up a bit for that added crunchy goodness!"

Preparation time: 10 minutes

Cooking time: 5 minutes

Servings: 4

Temperature: 360degreesF

Ingredients:

- One eggplant, peeled and sliced
- One flax-egg
- ½ cup cashew cheese
- 2 tbsp. almond milk
- 2 cups almond meal
- Cooking spray
- Black pepper
- Salt

Directions:

Take a bowl and add flax egg, salt, and pepper to it

Whisk it well

Take another bowl, mix cheese and panko, then stir

Dip eggplant fries in the flax egg mixture, coat in panko mix

Grease the Air Fryer basket using vegan cooking spray

Place the eggplant fries in it

Cook for 5 minutes at 400 degrees

Serve and enjoy!

Nutrition:

Calories: 162

Fat: 5g

Carbohoydrates: 7g

Protein: 6g

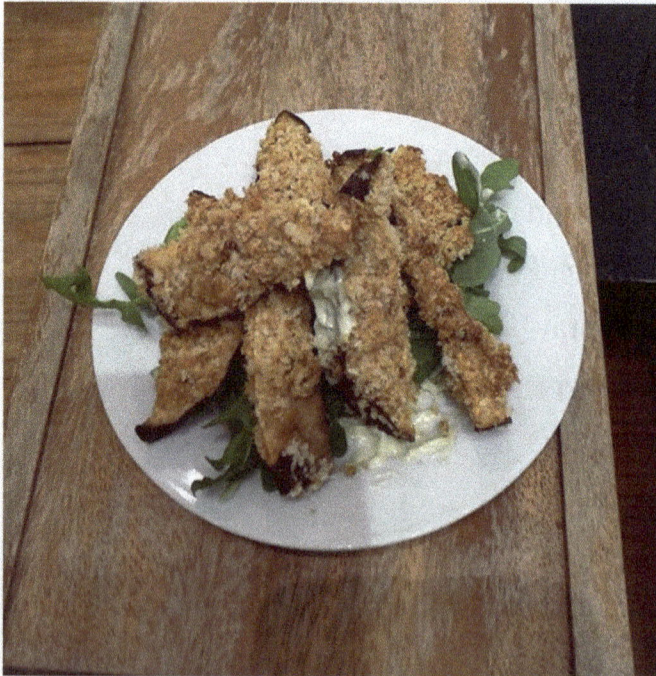

Crispy and Salty Tofu

"While many people don't like the flavour of normally prepared tofu, Air Drying them completely changes everything!"

Preparation time: 5 minutes

Cooking time: 15 minutes

Servings: 4

Temperature: 392degreesF

Ingredients:

- ¼ cup chickpea flour
- ¼ cup arrowroot
- 1 tsp. salt
- 1 tsp. garlic powder
- ½ tsp. black pepper
- One pack (15 ounces) tofu, firm
- Cooking spray as needed

Directions:

Preheat your Air Fryer 392 Degrees F

Take a medium-sized bowl and add flour, arrowroot, salt, garlic, pepper, and stir well

Cut tofu into cubes, transfer cubes into the flour mix

Toss well

Spray tofu with oil and transfer to Air Fryer cooking basket

Spray oil on top and cook for 8 minutes

Shake and toss well, fry for 7 minutes more

Serve and enjoy!

Nutrition:

Calories: 148

Fat: 5g

Carbohoydrates: 14g

Protein: 11g

Vegan Staples

Crumbed Tempeh

This vegan version of fish fingers is healthy and oil-free! Perfect for the kids, served with ketchup or mayo.

Preparation time: 5 minutes
Cooking time: 12 minutes
Servings: 2

Ingredients:
- 200g packet tempeh
- 3 - 4 tbsp. besan flour
- ½ tsp. of celery salt
- 1 tsp. smoked paprika
- ½ cup Panko breadcrumbs
- Almond Milk

Directions:
Slice up the tempeh in 1cm strips.
Mix the besan flour, celery salt and paprika.
Dip the tempeh strip into the almond milk, then coat with the flour mix.

Put the tempeh back into the milk and then coat with the breadcrumbs.

Sprinkle a little extra celery salt and cook at 180 degrees Celsius for 12 mins.

Nutrition:

Energy (calories): 235 kcal

Protein: 20.95 g

Fat: 11.62 g

Carbohydrates: 15.82 g

Fried Lasagna

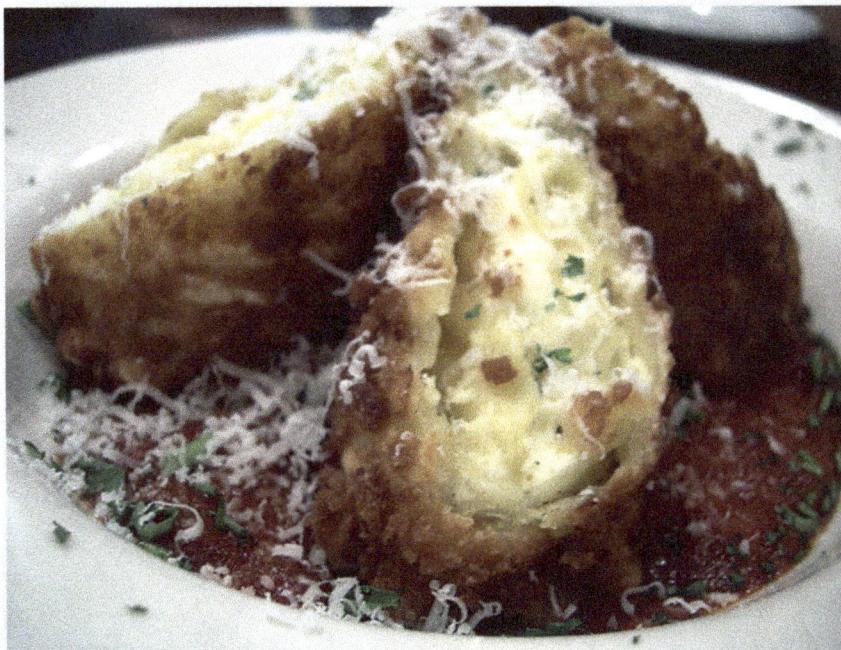

Tofu ricotta filled lasagna noodles coated in bread crumbs, and herbs feature hearty Italian flavours that truly delight. Serve alongside marinara sauce for a flavour explosion.

Preparation time: 15 minutes
Cooking time: 15 minutes
Servings: 2

Ingredients:

- 6 Lasagna sheets
- 4 oz. block extra-firm tofu
- 2 tbsp. Nutritional yeast
- Two cloves garlic
- 2 tbsp. lemon juice
- 2 tsp. Olive oil
- ½ tsp. salt
- A pinch of black pepper
- 1 cup vegan bread crumb s
- 1 cup almond milk
- 1 tsp. Apple cider vinegar
- ½ tsp. Garlic powder
- ½ tsp. Dried parsley
- ½ tsp. dried oregano

Directions:

Boil the lasagna sheets according to packet instructions and set aside.

Squeeze some liquid out of the tofu over the sink. It will crumble.

Add the crumbled tofu, Nutritional yeast, garlic, olive oil, lemon juice, salt and pepper to a food processor.

Pulse until everything comes together and is smooth, but with some texture.

Once the lasagna sheets are cool, take one sheet, pat it dry and place it flat on a plate. Spread the whole sheet with about 1-2 tbsp, of the tofu ricotta mixture. Spread evenly in a thin layer.

Fold one side part of the lasagna sheet to the center, and then fold the other side over.

Press down the end and seal in as much as possible.

Pour the almond milk and apple cider vinegar to one bowl, whisk and let sit for 1 minute to curdle slightly.

In another separate bowl, add the bread crumbs and dried herbs, stirring to combine.

Take one folded lasagna, dip it into the almond milk, and then put in the bread crumbs and coat thoroughly. Press the breadcrumbs gently onto the pasta, so they stick.

Place the lasagna pockets in the air fryer spray with cooking oil spray and air fry at 400 degrees Fahrenheit for 7-9 minutes. Flip them halfway through cooking and cook until they are brown and crispy. Enjoy!

Nutrition:
Energy (calories): 266 kcal
Protein: 16.16 g
Fat: 12.66 g
Carbohydrates: 24.26 g

Buffalo Tofu

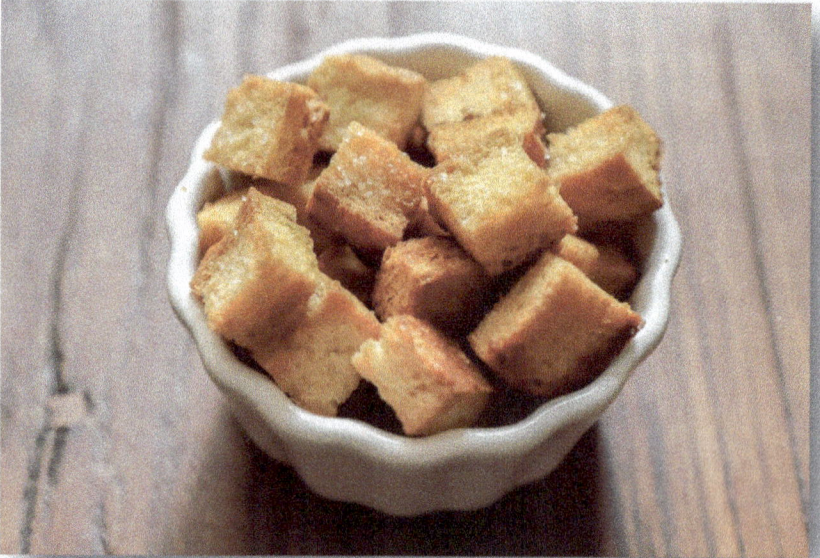

This 3-ingredient Buffalo tofu is a quick, easy and delicious snack! It cooks in under half an hour, so perfect for a movie night or game day.

Preparation time: 60 minutes
Cooking time: 20 minutes
Servings: 2

Ingredients:

- One block extra-firm tofu drained and pressed
- 1 cup hot sauce
- ¼ cup vegan butter, melted
- To Serve:
- Vegan ranch or blue cheese dressing

Directions:

Cut the tofu into squares.

Preheat and set the air fryer's temperature to 390 degrees Fahrenheit.

Whisk the hot sauce together with the melted butter to form the buffalo sauce.

Marinate the tofu in the buffalo sauce mixture for 30 - 60 minutes.

Once the air fryer is preheated, coat the basket lightly with cooking oil spray and use tongs and add the tofu to the air fryer basket. Reserve the marinade.

Air-fry for 20 - 30 minutes, checking and shaking the tofu after 10 minutes, and then each additional 5 minutes after that.

Check the tofu each time for the desired crispness.

Toss the tofu back into the reserved hot sauce and then transfer to a serving plate.

If desired, serve alongside vegan blue cheese or ranch dressing and enjoy!

Nutrition:

Energy (calories): 448 kcal

Protein: 24.74 g

Fat: 36.52 g

Carbohydrates: 13.3 g

Support for College Students

Nutritional Medicine Major